THE BIBLE CURE®

FOR

ARTHRITIS

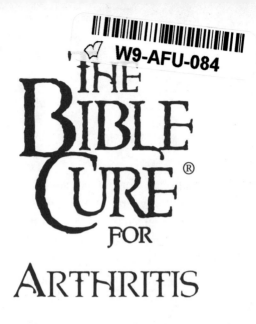

DON COLBERT, M.D.

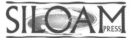

SILOAM PRESS

Living in Health—Body, Mind and Spirit

THE BIBLE CURE FOR ARTHRITIS
by Don Colbert, M.D.
Published by Siloam Press
A part of Strang Communications Company
600 Rinehart Road
Lake Mary, Florida 32746
www.siloampress.com

Unless otherwise noted, Scripture quotations are from the Holy Bible, New Living Translation, copyright © 1996. Used by permission of Tyndale House Publishers, Inc., Wheaton, IL 60189.

Scripture quotations marked KJV are from the King James Version of the Bible.

Library of Congress Catalog Card Number:
99-93491

International Standard Book Number:
0-88419-649-6

01 02 03 04   13 12 11 10 9
Printed in the United States of America

You Can
Overcome Arthritis

G od understands your pain and suffering. In fact, the Bible talks specifically about arthritis pain. This biblical songwriter may be echoing your feelings exactly when he wrote, "My life is poured out like water, and all my bones are out of joint. My heart is like wax, melting within me . . . I can count every bone in my body" (Ps. 22:14, 17). Not only does God understand your pain, but He has provided natural, medical and spiritual ways for you to overcome your pain and be healed.

Throughout this book you will learn how to care for your body, which is the temple of God's Spirit. (See 1 Corinthians 3:16–17.) God the Healer desires for you to be physically healthy so that you can enjoy life to its fullest and serve Him.

Are you suffering with *rheumatoid arthritis*—called an autoimmune disease because your symptoms are caused by your body's immune system attacking itself? Or have you been diagnosed with *osteoarthritis*—caused by the degeneration of your joints and the loss of cartilage? This Bible Cure booklet is designed to help you overcome your pain with good nutrition, exercise, prayer, Scripture and faith in Jesus Christ.

You are about to discover that sensitivity to certain chemicals and foods you eat can trigger arthritis symptoms. In fact, nightshade plants are suspected to trigger worst reactions.[1] Researchers have discovered that nightshade plants like potatoes, tomatoes, eggplants and peppers affect over one-third of those who suffer from rheumatoid arthritis. Already you have learned one simple thing you can do through God's Bible cure that may help relieve rheumatoid arthritis—decrease your intake of nightshade plants.

We ingest thousands of chemical additives every day in our foods. Our bodies may be highly allergic or sensitive to many of those additives. Throughout this book you will discover what foods to avoid while learning what foods you can and should eat.

A BIBLE CURE PRAYER
FOR YOU

Almighty God, help me to develop both knowledge and wisdom about natural foods that will strengthen my body and not cause allergic reactions. Give me the time and patience to carefully read about and then use the right foods and supplements suggested in this book so that I will overcome the pain of arthritis. Amen.

As you shop for food, ask the Holy Spirit to guide you and give you both the wisdom and desire to read labels.

Arthritis pain is not new. Did you know that arthritis is one of the earliest documented afflictions in history? Scientists have discovered evidence of arthritis in the bones of mummies from the pyramids of ancient Egypt. But this ancient disease has a remedy older than history—the Ancient of Days who is God the Healer. For millennia people have suffered unnecessarily. God has not only provided many natural ways for you to be relieved of arthritic pain, but He has also provided supernatural healing for your body through trusting His Word and drawing near to Him. Listen to His promise:

> If you will listen carefully to the voice of the LORD your God and do what is right in his sight, obeying his commands and laws, then I will not make you suffer the diseases I sent on the Egyptians; for I am the LORD who heals you.
>
> —EXODUS 15:26

Through prayer and Scripture, God is speaking to you. This book will be a guide for you to hear His voice and to discern His Bible cure for your arthritis. In this book, you will

uncover God's divine
plan of health for body, soul and spirit
through modern medicine, good nutrition
and the medicinal power
of Scripture and prayer.

Throughout this book are key scriptures that will help you focus on the healing power of God through the Bible. These ancient texts will guide your prayers and direct your thoughts toward God's plan of divine health for you in preventing or battling arthritis.

In this Bible Cure booklet, you will discover how to overcome the pain of arthritis through chapters on:

Don't give up. Keep pushing through for your Bible cure for arthritis. It is my prayer that these practical suggestions for healing, prayer, nutrition and fitness will bring healing to your life. I trust that they will build hope within you and strengthen your faith as God strengthens you to overcome arthritis.

—Don Colbert, M.D.

A BIBLE CURE PRAYER
FOR YOU

Almighty God, I pray for Your wisdom and knowledge to do those things that You direct so that I may overcome arthritis. Help me to discover any foods that contain substances or toxins that are triggering allergic responses in my body. I speak to the swelling and pain in my joints and bones and command it to go, in Jesus' name. I thank You, Lord, for Your healing anointing to straighten and strengthen my whole skeletal system. I ask for Your wisdom to empower me to learn both your natural and supernatural ways for victory over arthritis. By faith I claim Your promise as my Healer. Cleanse my body from this disease through the shed blood of Jesus Christ. Amen.

Chapter 1

Overcoming Arthritis

W hile there are many different forms of arthritis, in this book we will be discussing two of the main forms of arthritis—osteoarthritis and rheumatoid arthritis. You will learn important facts and information that will encourage you to take positive steps toward overcoming arthritis. You will also discover vital scriptures throughout this book that will build in you a spiritual and mental attitude to empower you to overcome fear, depression, anxiety and discouragement as you win the battle against arthritis.

One of your first steps toward feeling better is understanding the difference between rheumatoid arthritis and osteoarthritis. Let's contrast these two forms of arthritis, and then we will walk through some initial, positive steps you can take naturally and spiritually to uncover your Bible cure prescription for rheumatoid arthritis and osteo-arthritis.

Which Kind of Arthritis Are You Overcoming?

Below you will discover the differences between rheumatoid arthritis and osteoarthritis. I have identified for you the commonly recognized symptoms of both diseases.

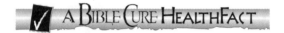

Rheumatoid Arthritis

- Is an autoimmune disease that often afflicts those from ages 25–50
- Usually occurs in younger adults, but it can attack children, even infants
- Usually affects joints on both sides of the body (e.g. both knees)
- Causes redness, warmth and swelling of many joints and attacks many joints, often the small joints of the hands, feet, ankles, knees and elbows
- Causes major fatigue of your whole body
- Causes prolonged morning stiffness

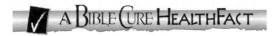
Osteoarthritis

- Caused by the wear and tear of cartilage
- Usually affects people after age 40
- Affects isolated joints, or joints on only one side of the body at first
- Causes discomfort in the joints but does not usually cause swelling; particularly affects the weight-bearing joints like the hips and knees
- Does not usually cause fatigue
- Causes brief morning stiffness

HEALTHFACT HEALTHFACT HEALTHFACT HEALTHFACT HEALTHFACT HEALTHFACT HEALTHFACT

Do You Have Osteoarthritis?

Osteoarthritis is by far the most common form of arthritis. It is also termed degenerative joint disease. Osteoarthritis is most often characterized by joint pain. The joint pain is due to a gradual loss of cartilage and degeneration of the joint. Over forty million Americans suffer from osteoarthritis. Osteoarthritis primarily affects the larger weight-bearing joints. Approximately 80 percent of Americans over the age of fifty suffer from arthritis. There are two main forms of osteoarthritis, primary and secondary.

Primary osteoarthritis usually begins after the age of forty-five, affecting the fingers, neck, lower back, knees and hips. While the cause is unknown, we do know that obese individuals tend to develop it more commonly. As you gain weight, the pressure on the weight-bearing joints such as the hips and knees increases dramatically. When an obese patient runs or jumps, the pressure on the joints can be as much as ten times a person's body weight. In other words, if a two-hundred-fifty-pound man jumped down off of a ladder, the pressure on his hips and knees could be as much as a ton. Is there any wonder why patients who are obese are becoming crippled with osteoarthritis?

Secondary osteoarthritis is simply due to trauma. I commonly see ex-football players in my practice who are crippled with osteoarthritis, especially in the fingers and the knees due to repeated trauma of these joints. Weightlifters commonly get arthritis in their shoulders and knees due to repetitive trauma to these joints. Tennis players commonly get arthritis in their dominant shoulder, whereas golfers commonly get arthritis in their lower back. Continually moving these joints in the same way causes this arthritis, which can eventually lead to chronic trauma and then to degeneration of the joint.

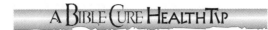
A Self-Test for Osteoarthritis

The following symptoms are common to those suffering from osteoarthritis. Check the symptoms you have. If you have checked many of the symptoms below, check with your physician and a nutritional doctor for direction and guidance.

- ❑ I have early morning stiffness.
- ❑ I am stiff following periods of rest.
- ❑ My pain worsens with joint use.
- ❑ I have loss of joint function.
- ❑ My joints seem tender.
- ❑ My joints creak and crack with movement.
- ❑ My mobility is restricted.

Factory workers and construction workers also commonly develop osteoarthritis due to the repetitive nature of their work. For instance, a worker on an assembly line doing the same job over and over usually will develop arthritis in his fingers, whereas a carpet layer will develop it in his knees and hands.

A sheet-metal worker came as a patient to our office with swollen finger joints in both hands. He claimed that for the past thirty years he had been working with a nail gun that drives nails through metal. This worker is on the way to overcoming arthritis, and you can, too.

Do You Have Rheumatoid Arthritis?

Rheumatoid arthritis is different from osteo-arthritis. It affects approximately ten million Americans, striking women three times more often than men. While osteoarthritis is age-related, rheumatoid arthritis is an autoimmune disease; the body is actually attacking itself. It not only affects the joints, but it also affects the entire body due to chronic inflammation. The joints affected are usually swollen, tender, warm to touch and quite stiff.

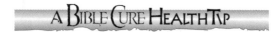

A BIBLE CURE HEALTH TIP

A Self-Test for Rheumatoid Arthritis

Check off the following items that apply to you:
- ❑ My age is between 25 and 50.
- ❑ Pain and swelling in my joints developed within just a few weeks or months.
- ❑ The joints on both sides of my body are affected.
- ❑ My joints are swollen, red and warm.
- ❑ I am experiencing general feelings of fatigue and sickness.

❑ I have lost weight.
❑ I often have a fever.
❑ I am stiff in the mornings.
❑ I have been experiencing major fatigue.

(If you are experiencing the symptoms described above, consult with your physician.)

Let's stop right now and address the symptom of fatigue. When you are tired and exhausted from pain, it seems impossible to maintain a positive outlook. You may feel discouraged, but God knows your circumstance; He will give you strength and rest. Take a moment right now to read aloud and meditate on these guidelines from Scripture for rest, and then pray the Bible cure prayer.

Those who live in the shelter of the Most High will find rest in the shadow of the Almighty. This I declare of the LORD: He alone is my refuge, my place of safety; he is my God, and I am trusting him. For he will rescue you from every trap and protect you from the fatal plague. He will shield you with his wings. He will shelter you with his feathers. His faithful promises are your armor and protection. Do not be afraid of the terrors of the night, nor fear the dangers of the day, nor dread the plague that stalks in darkness, nor the disaster that strikes at midday. Though a thousand fall at your side, though ten thousand are dying around you, these evils will not touch you.

—PSALM 91:1–7

A BIBLE CURE PRAYER
FOR YOU

Almighty God, I seek the shelter of Your wings. I long to rest in You. Take away my fear and pain in the night, and grant me Your hope and peace. In Jesus' name, I come against the evil attack of arthritis and claim You as my Healer, my Rock and my Deliverer. I praise You now, Lord, for the healing You provided through the shed blood of Jesus Christ. I ask, Lord Jesus, that as the Prince of Peace You fill my spirit, soul and body with Your healing rest. Amen.

Taking the Bible cure spiritual steps that I recommend throughout this book will open your life to God's healing touch. He has not left you, and He will not forsake you. God will make a way for you both naturally and spiritually to overcome arthritis. Now let's discuss some of the natural ways you can overcome this physical attack!

In the next few chapters, you will discover natural and spiritual steps you can take to feel better and overcome either rheumatoid arthritis or osteoarthritis. But first, I want to encourage you to begin laying a spiritual foundation that will build your faith and hope as you do all you can do to overcome arthritis and seek God to do the rest.

Overcoming Arthritis Spiritually

Taking the natural steps outlined in this book will help you feel better physically, but there is still more that you can do to overcome arthritis and the discouragement that comes with it. Your most important weapon in this battle is prayer. God can supernaturally heal your rheumatoid arthritis or your osteoarthritis as you pray, learn His Word and seek Him.

Prayer works.

In the Bible, Hezekiah, a king of Israel, discovered that God heals in response to prayer. The prophet Isaiah came to Hezekiah with the dreaded word that the king would die (2 Kings 20:1). You may have received a discouraging word from your doctor. People around you may have told you about the suffering they have experienced with arthritis. You don't have to accept that word as the final word on your future health! If you are to grow stronger spiritually to overcome this disease, you must first strengthen your faith and pray with boldness.

Stop listening to negative reports.

Once you know the facts about your arthritis, don't allow your mind to become overwhelmed with thoughts about how bad this disease can become. Instead, begin taking positive steps in the natural and spiritual realms to strengthen your spirit and your body. A strong spirit

> *My life is poured out like water, and all my bones are out of joint . . . I can count every bone in my body. . . . O Lord, do not stay away! You are my strength; come quickly to my aid!*
> —PSALM 22:14–19

will help your body fight and overcome disease.

Whose report will you believe? Doctors can give you test results and inform you about the facts of past statistics, studies and symptoms associated with rheumatoid arthritis. But physicians cannot predict or determine your future. Your future is in God's hands. In 2 Kings 20, Hezekiah refused to accept the prophet's negative report as the final word about his illness. He took a positive step in response to a negative report—he prayed!

Pray in faith.

Hezekiah " . . . turned his face to the wall and prayed to the LORD, 'Remember, O LORD, how I have always tried to be faithful to you and do what is pleasing in your sight.' Then he broke down and wept bitterly" (2 Kings 20:2–3).

God heard Hezekiah's prayer and healed him! Read what God said in response to Hezekiah's prayer: "I have heard your prayer and seen your tears. I will heal you, and three days from now you will get out of bed and go to the Temple of the LORD" (2 Kings 20:5).

Surround yourself with prayer warriors.

Do not surround yourself with negative people

who only give you sympathy and talk about how bad things are now and how much worse they will get. We all know these people. They seem to be able to quench your faith with one word. My advice: Stay away from doomsayers. The Bible says:

> Oh, the joys of those who do not follow the advice of the wicked, or stand around with sinners, or join in with scoffers. But they delight in doing everything the LORD wants; day and night they think about his law. They are like trees planted along the riverbank, bearing fruit each season without fail. Their leaves never wither, and in all they do, they prosper.
>
> —PSALM 1:1–3

Surround yourself with people who will pray with you and agree in faith for your healing. Jesus the Healer makes this promise: "I tell you this: Whatever you prohibit on earth is prohibited in heaven, and whatever you allow on earth is allowed in heaven. I also tell you this: If two of you agree down here on earth concerning anything you ask, my Father in heaven will do it for you" (Matt. 18:18–19).

How do you agree in prayer with friends for your healing? Surround yourself with people of faith, not of doubt. Ask them to join you in praying this prayer of agreement.

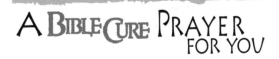

A BIBLE CURE PRAYER
FOR YOU

Lord Jesus Christ, our Healer, we agree together in Your name for overcoming arthritis. We prohibit the attack of arthritis and agree for healing from pain, swollen joints and all the attacks of arthritis against the temple of the Holy Spirit. We declare healing from arthritis, because by Your strips we are healed. We break the curse of every negative report and choose to believe the good report that You have forgiven all our sins and healed all our diseases. In Jesus' name, Amen.

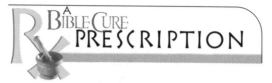

A BIBLE CURE PRESCRIPTION

As you have begun understanding arthritis, summarize what you have learned about:

Osteoarthritis

_____

_____

Rheumatoid arthritis

_____

_____

Check the spiritual steps you will take:

❏ Stop dwelling on negative reports and your pain.

❏ Seek God through His Word and through prayer for your healing.

❏ Find friends filled with hope and faith who will agree with you in prayer for your healing.

❏ Agree with others in faith through prayer for God's healing power to remove your pain and heal arthritis.

Chapter 2

Overcoming Arthritis With Proper Nutrition

We are told in the Bible that our bodies are the temples of the Holy Spirit. "Don't you realize that all of you together are the temple of God and that the Spirit of God lives in you? God will bring ruin upon anyone who ruins this temple. For God's temple is holy, and you Christians are that temple" (1 Cor. 3:16–17). We honor God when we maintain our bodies physically so that we may serve Him and others. One way we take care of our temples is through proper nutrition.

Two essential steps for preventing and combating osteoarthritis are drinking lots of water and eating right—proper nutrition. You can begin them today and immediately feel better! We will also learn some spiritual steps necessary for over-coming osteoarthritis.

Take Care of Your Cartilage

The Bible says that we are fearfully and wonderfully made (Ps. 139). One of the marvels of your body is cartilage. God created the cartilage in your joints to be a remarkable shock absorber for your body. If you take care of your cartilage by drinking lots of water and losing weight, which we will discuss later in this book, then you will be taking giant strides in successfully overcoming osteoarthritis.

There are many different types of joints in the human body, but there are three main classes—the fixed joints, the slightly moveable joints and the highly moveable joints. The highly moveable joints are most commonly affected with os-teoarthritis. These include the elbows, knees, shoulders, hips, fingers, toes, ankles and wrists. Each of these joints is covered with articular car-tilage. This cartilage is very smooth and shiny and is very similar in appearance to the cartilage on the drumstick of a chicken. It is bluish-white in color and is extremely smooth and slick. It is ap-proximately eight times as slick as ice.

In trying to imagine how smooth this normal cartilage is, recall one cold winter when the roads were iced over and your boots also had ice on them. It was sleeting, and when your wet, iced-over boot hit the iced-over pavement, you went sliding. Well, the joint surface is eight times slicker than that iced surface on which you slipped.

Cartilage is approximately 80 percent water, and the remainder of the cartilage is made up of proteoglycans, collagen and chondrocytes. Cartilage serves as your body's shock absorber by cushioning the joints, and it prevents damage to the joint during different activities.

> Don't turn away from me in my time of distress. Bend down your ear and answer me quickly when I call to you, for my days disappear like smoke, and my bones burn like red-hot coals.
> —PSALM 102:2–3

Cartilage has no blood vessels in it; it depends on fluid exchange in order to be nourished. Collagen is made up of amino acids that form protein chains. The collagen actually provides the strength and elasticity to the cartilage. Collagen acts like reinforcement beams that hold the proteoglycans in place.

Proteoglycans, on the other hand, are made of protein and sugar. They encircle the collagen fibers, forming a dense, water-loving, filler-like material in between the strong strands of collagen. They hold the collagen threads together, acting like a type of mortar. The cartilage gets both its shape and strength from the proteoglycans.

In high school I played basketball, and I wore Converse tennis shoes that had almost no cushioning present. Today, I wear Nike Air shoes that have an air bubble that extends from the heel to the toes. This air pocket creates a cushion for the foot that allows me to walk on hard surfaces without any discomfort.

Your cartilage also serves just like a shock absorber. When it is healthy we can engage in practically any sport or activity without pain. However, when the cartilage becomes thin and worn, we then develop pain with certain activities, which is analogous to the Converse tennis shoes that I wore in high school, which had little to no cushioning.

If the cells in your cartilage start dying due to toxicity, poor nutrition or systemic disease process, then the cartilage is unable to be adequately repaired. Your cartilage framework then begins to splinter. The cartilage begins to crack and break off, and this leads to joint degeneration.

As the cartilage wears, enzymes are also leaked into the cartilage, which actually destroy more of the collagen and more of the proteoglycans. It then becomes a vicious cycle of joint destruction and increased joint pain.

Eventually the cartilage becomes so thin and worn that it actually wears through, and the bone is exposed. When this occurs, it is very difficult to repair the cartilage. The body forms an inferior form of cartilage called *fibro-cartilage*. This layer covers the bone. However, it only has a very short life span, so it is constantly being worn out. When this cartilage is finally gone, bone rubs upon bone, which causes severe pain. The bones also become extremely inflamed, and fluid from your cartilage leaking into the damaged bones causes even further damage.

As you can see, this is a vicious cycle that continues to get worse and worse. Therefore, it is important to identify this disease early and to begin aggressive lifestyle and nutritional management as soon as possible. To keep your cartilage healthy, begin today to drink lots of water and eat right through proper nutrition.

Step 1: Drink lots of water—proper hydration.

Water is also extremely important in preventing osteoarthritis. Since cartilage is composed of approximately 80 percent water, I believe it is critically important to drink at least two quarts of water per day. Cartilage is similar to a sponge. The spongy cartilage soaks up synovial fluid when the joint is at rest. However, when pressure is placed on the joint, synovial fluid is squeezed out. The synovial fluid thus squeezes in and out of the cartilage with rest and activity. It is therefore critical to have sufficient water intake in order to have adequate synovial fluid.

A BIBLE CURE PRAYER
FOR YOU

Almighty God, I thank You for the healing, refreshing and cleansing properties of Your wondrous creation—water. Use the water I drink to refresh my body and help the cartilage in my joints heal. Father, fill me with the living water of Your Spirit so that my faith will be renewed, my spirit refreshed and my hope in You restored. In Jesus' name, amen.

As mentioned before, the proteoglycans of the cartilage are the primary portion of the cartilage that holds the water. With osteoarthritis, the cartilage eventually dries out and thins. This then leads to cracking and further destruction of the cartilage.

Step 2: Eat right—proper nutrition.

You can avoid certain foods that will actually trigger inflammation. And you can eat other foods that will actually help strengthen and renew your cartilage. Let's explore how proper nutrition will help you win the battle against arthritis.

Avoid foods with arachidonic acid. Arachidonic acid is a fatty acid that is found primarily in saturated fats and animal products. These products include red meat, pork, egg yolks, poultry and all dairy products except for nonfat dairy products. Arachidonic acid causes production of a dangerous form of prostaglandin, which actually promotes inflammation.

Avoid foods rich in omega-6 fatty acids. Since inflammation is the main characteristic of rheumatoid arthritis, it is essential to control inflammation. I believe dietary factors such as decreasing or eliminating dangerous fats and taking in the good fats on a daily basis are essential in controlling inflammation.

As much as possible, avoid oils rich in omega-6 fatty acids, which include safflower, corn and sunflower oils, margarine and most other kinds of plant oils. Also avoid all fried foods.

Use extra-virgin olive oil and other foods that are high in monounsaturated fats, which include almonds, avocados, macadamia nuts and canola oil.

The Mediterranean diet eaten by those living in the regions around the Mediterranean Sea is rich in olive oil. The Bible reveals both the natural and spiritual dynamic of olives and olive oil. In addition to its dietary and ceremonial uses, olive oil was also used medicinally. Beyond its natural healing properties, the Bible also instructs us to be anointed with oil for healing. (See James 5:14.)

I would encourage you to call upon your spiritual elders and have them anoint you with oil and pray for your healing. This will build your faith, strengthen your hope and impart God's healing power upon you.

Anointing With Oil

Not only do the substances in olive oil help you physically, but there is a spiritual lesson for being anointed with oil when you are sick. Speak aloud, memorize and meditate upon this Scripture. Then ask your elders to anoint you with oil and pray.

> Are any among you sick? They should call for the elders of the church and have them pray over them, anointing them with oil in the name of the Lord.
>
> —JAMES 5:14

Jesus, anoint me with the oil of Your Spirit so that I may be healed physically. In Your name I rebuke the attacks of arthritis on my body and seek for Your healing power to touch and heal my cartilage, joints, bones and digestive system in Jesus' name. Amen.

Eat foods rich in omega-3 fatty acids. EPA, which is an omega-3 fatty acid found primarily in fatty fish and marine plants, is very effective in reducing inflammation. Fatty fish include salmon, mackerel, herring, tuna, sardines and trout. One should have at least three to five servings of fatty fish per week. If unable to eat these fish on a weekly basis, take omega-3 fatty acid supplements, approximately three capsules with each meal. One should also take digestive enzymes with these.

The Bible describes fish with fins and scales as being clean. (See Leviticus 11:9.) The Hebrews would often eat fish on the Sabbath. This could include all the fish mentioned above, which are rich in omega-3 fatty acids. Those foods clean in the Bible cure are pure and healthy for us. God has provided healthy foods for you to eat and enjoy that will help your body heal and keep you in divine health.

Revelations From Arthritis Research

Epidemiological studies of Eskimos in Greenland have demonstrated the potential anti-inflammatory effects of omega-3 fatty acids, which are plentiful in their high-seafood diet. The Eskimos' prevalence of chronic infammatory diseases is lower than that of inhabitants of Western countries.[1]

Researchers at Tufts University in Boston found

that the B_6 levels in twenty-six rheumatoid arthritis patients were lower than the B_6 levels in healthy subjects. Foods rich in B_6 include brewer's yeast, brown rice, whole wheat, soybeans, rye, lentils, sunflower seeds, hazelnuts, alfalfa, salmon, wheat germ, tuna, bran, walnuts, peas and beans.[2]

Overcoming Rheumatoid Arthritis Through Proper Nutrition

While rheumatoid arthritis affects approximately ten million Americans each year and is often seen as more difficult to treat than osteoarthritis, good news has emerged both from research and faith. In this section, you will discover how eliminating foods you are allergic to will immediately help you feel better. And you will uncover the power of prayer and God's healing power for rheumatoid arthritis. Don't be discouraged. Through God's guidance and healing touch you can overcome arthritis and begin feeling relief and rest from your pain.

As I mentioned earlier in this book, studies have confirmed that many of the symptoms related to rheumatoid arthritis may be linked to food allergies. You can begin to feel better, reduce your pain and begin experiencing God's healing power this very moment. How? Let me share with you some simple natural and spiritual steps.

Step 1. Eliminate foods to which you may be allergic from your diet.

Many people with rheumatoid arthritis have food allergies or sensitivities. Many common foods may trigger the symptoms of rheumatoid arthritis.

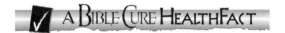

Foods That Trigger Rheumatoid Arthritic Reactions

- Corn
- Pork
- Rye
- Beef
- Oranges
- Milk and dairy products
- Nightshade plants, which include tomatoes, eggplant, potatoes and bell peppers

- Wheat
- Oats
- Eggs
- Coffee
- Grapefruit

HEALTHFACT HEALTHFACT HEALTHFACT HEALTHFACT HEALTHFACT HEALTHFACT HEALTHFACT

You can perform a food elimination diet. Here's how you do it. First, for two weeks stop eating the foods I have listed in the box on this page. Then add one of the foods to your diet for a week. If you do not experience any increase in your rheumatoid arthritis symptoms, then that food is probably safe for you to continue eating. If you have an increase in pain, swelling, redness and warmth in your joints, then the food you added is possibly dangerous for you to eat. You may well be allergic or sensitive to it.

In the Bible, fasting serves spiritual purposes, but it can also have tremendous natural benefits for your body. If you have been suffering from food allergies, fast for a few days with filtered or distilled water. One may also have white rice since this is very hypoallergenic compared to most other foods.

> *Dry bones, listen to the word of the LORD! . . . Look! I am going to breathe into you and make you live again! I will put flesh and muscles on you and cover you with skin. I will put breath into you, and you will come to life. Then you will know that I am the LORD.*
> —EZEKIEL 37:4–6

I have helped many of my arthritic patients who also have food allergies with the N.A.E.T. desensitization program. This therapy is used by physicians with extensive training in nutritional therapy. It is a natural, drugless, painless and noninvasive method of elimination of allergies one at a time.[3]

Step 2. Help your intestines heal through proper nutrition.

A healthy intestinal tract will greatly improve how you feel physically and will help reduce your arthritic symptoms. Proper absorption in your intestinal tract will insure that the nutrients you need for healing will reach your bones and joints. Reducing the inflammation of your digestive tract will also help relieve some of the painful symptoms you may be experiencing.

An important initial step for you to take that will help overcome rheumatoid arthritis is to improve the condition of your digestive tract. Then it can heal and maintain its normal permeability, thus allowing essential vitamins and minerals to reach your joints and bones with their healing properites.

> *At least I can take comfort in this: Despite the pain, I have not denied the words of the Holy One.*
> —Job 6:10

The intestinal lining has one of the fastest growth rates of any tissue in the body other than the cornea. A completely new lining is formed every three to six days as the old cells slough off. You can help your irritated intestine heal naturally through God-given substances, such as those listed below.

Fish oil, evening primrose oil and black currant oil: Essential fatty acids such as fish oil and evening primrose oil (one or two capsules three times a day with meals) and black currant oil (one capsule three times a day with meals) help maintain normal intestinal permeability. Talk about tart, currants are mouth-puckering, which is why they are rarely eaten just out of your hand. Here are some palatable ways to prepare currants if you want to get their beneficial, healing effects without taking black currant oil capsules.

- Like cranberries, currants make a perfect sauce for livening up meat dishes. They're slightly sweeter than cranberries, however, so you'll want to add a combination of red, white and black currants.
- Putting currants in fruit salads will add a tangy taste. For an even prettier plate, add a combination of red, white and black currants.[4]

A high-fiber diet: A high-fiber diet will also improve intestinal permeability and help you overcome rheumatoid arthritis. There are many different forms of fiber, which include psyllium, oat bran, rice bran, ground flaxseeds, guar gum and modified citrus pectin. Find your favorite form of fiber, and take it on a daily basis. I personally prefer fresh ground flaxseeds. However, you could also use over-the-counter psyllium products such as Perdiem Fiber, Metamucil or oat bran.

If you have rheumatoid arthritis, see a nutritional doctor and have a comprehensive digestive stool analysis performed. To improve digestion, you may need to take betaine HCL and pepsin along with pancreatic enzymes. Thoroughly chew your food and mix it well with saliva; do not wash the food down with fluids. Again, a nutritional doctor will help to initiate a program to improve your digestion and intestinal permeability.

Conclusion

We have explored together the essential steps you can take naturally to overcome arthritis through proper nutrition. As you drink lots of water, eat right and avoid those foods that may trigger arthritic inflammation in your body, you can also take spiritual steps that will further your success in overcoming arthritis.

Begin to thank God for all the foods He has provided to help your body overcome arthritis. Ask His Spirit to guide you as you shop to select those foods that are best for you. Keep in your house only those foods that will help you; do not even have in the pantry those which may cause arthritic inflammation. Then you eliminate the temptation to eat the wrong thing. Finally, pray that God's Spirit will completely heal your intestines so that all the nutrition your joints need will be properly digested and taken speedily by your circulatory system immediately to your joints and bones.

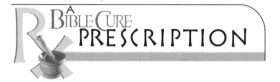

Overcoming Arthritis With Proper Nutrition

If you have osteoarthritis, check the steps you will take:

- ❏ Drink lots of water.
- ❏ Avoid foods with arachidonic acid.
- ❏ Avoid foods rich in omega-6 fatty acids. Use extra-virgin olive oil instead.
- ❏ Eat foods rich in omega-3 fatty acids.

If you have rheumatoid arthritis, check the steps you will take:

- ❏ Eliminate foods to which you are allergic.
- ❏ Help your intestines heal using fish oil, evening primrose oil or black currant oil.
- ❏ Maintain a high-fiber diet.

Check the spiritual steps you will take:

- ❏ Seek God's guidance in selecting the right foods to eat.
- ❏ Ask God to help you avoid even shopping for foods to which you are allergic.
- ❏ Pray for wisdom in caring for your body with proper nutrition.

Chapter 3

Overcoming Arthritis With Vitamins and Supplements

God's wonder substances for overcoming arthritis include vitamins and supplements. Of course, these natural substances are often found in nutritious foods; they may also be taken as supplements. God has created natural ways in our food and water to provide disease prevention and healing. But often our diets don't provide sufficient quantities of vital nutrients. That's why supplements are important. God gives us the responsibility to know how to care for our bodies naturally as well as how to apply His Word and pray spiritually for health.

Through these pages you will learn about God's natural wonders for overcoming arthritis. Whenever you encounter a Bible cure verse from

Scripture, take a moment to read it aloud, and then pray and ask God to empower you to apply both the scripture and all that you are learning in your lifestyle.

Fighting Osteoarthritis

Vitamins C and E. When considering God's natural substances, we must first turn to His awesome vitamins C and E. Antioxidant vitamins such as vitamin C and vitamin E may decrease cartilage loss. It may also slow down progression of osteoarthritis.

Vitamin C and E work synergistically, and they both protect against the breakdown of cartilage. They may actually help form cartilage. Take 800 International Units of natural vitamin E a day. You should also take at least 3,000 milligrams of vitamin C a day. I personally prefer the effervescent vitamin C known as Emergen-C.

Antioxidants like vitamins C and E are powerful agents that prevent oxidation caused by free radicals in our bodies. Free radicals are defective molecules that damage cells in our bodies.

God's wonder agents for helping our cells fight free radicals are antioxidants. Antioxidants are extremely important in strengthening our immune systems and helping our bodies overcome diseases like cancer, heart disease and arthritis.

Take a multivitamin. A comprehensive multivitamin is necessary in order to have proper amounts of vitamins and minerals that are required for both the manufacture and maintenance of cartilage. The vitamins should contain adequate levels of the minerals zinc, copper and boron, and also adequate levels of pantothenic acid, vitamin B_6 and vitamin A.

SAM-e. You might consider taking SAM-e, which is an amino acid that increases cartilage formation. While it is expensive, 200–400 milligrams of SAM-e two to three times a day may be effective in the manufacture of cartilage.

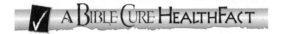

A BIBLE CURE HEALTHFACT

Taking S-Adenosylmethionine (SAM-e)

SAM-e is effective in a variety of metabolic pathways. It is especially effective in transferring carbons from one molecule to another.

Absorption/Storage, Dosage/Toxicity: The average amount recommended is 400 milligrams a day. Before taking product, you are advised to consult with a trained health care professional.

Deficiency: If there is an insufficient amount of methionine, then a deficiency in SAM-e may result.

Common Uses: Migraine headaches, depression, osteoarthritis and liver complications may all be treated with the use of SAM-e.

Precautions: Those suffering from manic depression should not take SAM-e. Gastrointestinal upset may be experienced. Consult a physician if pregnant or if symptoms of nausea, diarrhea or dizziness last more than a week or if new symptoms appear.[1]

HEALTHFACT HEALTHFACT HEALTHFACT HEALTHFACT HEALTHFACT HEALTHFACT HEALTHFACT

MSM. MSM (methylsulfanomethane) is another nutrient that may be effective in preventing or treating osteoarthritis. It contains high amounts of sulfur. Sulfur is an essential nutrient and is found in garlic, onions and cabbage. Healthy cartilage needs adequate sulfur. I recommend 500 milligrams of MSM, two to three tablets, three times a day.

Glucosamine sulfate—treating osteoarthritis naturally

In conventional medicine, the common treatment of osteoarthritis is the use of nonsteroidal anti-inflammatory drugs (NSAIDs), such as ibuprofen and naproxen. NSAIDs work by blocking the production of certain prostaglandins that cause inflammation and pain.

While these anti-inflammatory medications help reduce some of your inflammation and pain, they also have many side effects that can be quite serious, including gastrointestinal bleeding (especially from stomach ulcers). Research has actually shown that long-term use of anti-inflammatory medications may impair healing of the joints. This may further damage the cartilage. God has actually provided a natural way for the treatment of inflammation and pain in your joints.

In God's creation, the lowly crab is linked to osteoarthritis through a God-created wonder substance found in the exoskeleton of arthropods like the crab— glucosamine sulfate. Studies have shown that patients can have as

> *Turn to me and have mercy on me, for I am alone and in deep distress. My problems go from bad to worse. Oh, save me from them all! Feel my pain and see my trouble. Forgive all my sins.*
> —PSALM 25:15–18

much as a 71 percent improvement using this awesome substance from God's natural created order.[2]

Glucosamine sulfate is a compound composed of glucose, glutamine (which is an amino acid) and sulfur. Glucosamine sulfate is used to manufacture proteoglycans. The proteoglycans are the mortar that holds the collagen together and retains the water in the cartilage. Due to the tremendous water content of the proteoglycans, the cartilage absorbs water like a sponge when pressure is released from a joint, and the cartilage squeezes that water out when pressure is put on the joint.

Glucosamine also may trigger the cells in your cartilage (chondrocytes) to produce more proteoglycans and collagen. In addition, glucosamine may help to repair damaged cartilage. Therefore, over time, supplementation with glucosamine sulfate will help to relieve pain from osteoarthritis. Glucosamine sulfate is also able to inhibit enzymes that break down the cartilage. So glucosamine is used to make more proteoglycans in collagen, to repair damaged cartilage and to inhibit enzymes that would normally break down cartilage.

Studies have compared glucosamine to ibuprofen. Ibuprofen proved to be more effective in the first couple of weeks of therapy. But after the second week on, the glucosamine group and the ibuprofen group were practically even in pain-relief effectiveness.[3]

Anti-inflammatory medications and pain relievers will mask the pain of osteoarthritis. As a result, you may feel that you can go out and exercise without any pain. However, in doing so, you may actually be doing more damage to the joint since the anti-inflammatory or the pain medicine is only masking the pain. Glucosamine sulfate, however, is actually supplying the proteoglycans, thus helping to repair the cartilage. More water is put into the cartilage. Therefore, after being on glucosamine sulfate for approximately a month, you should have minimal pain while exercising as compared to masked pain with an anti-inflammatory pain reliever.

Glucosamine sulfate is a wonderful, God-created substance that can help your body fight back against osteoarthritis.

Anti-inflammatory supplements

As the joints in the body become progressively damaged by osteoarthritis, inflammation occurs. Inflammation is simply the body's natural response to damaged tissue. The inflammation then leads to warm, swollen, tender and stiff joints. When the tissue is damaged, the body sends white blood cells to these areas of inflammation. The white blood cells produce leukotrienes and other products of inflammation, which thus cause more inflammation and create a vicious cycle.

If your osteoarthritis has reached the stage of chronic inflammation characterized by symptoms of swelling, stiffness, warmth and pain, then you should immediately begin a diet of anti-inflammatory supplements.

Flaxseed oil is plant oil that also helps to reduce inflammation. You may need to take extra zinc with flaxseed oil, so check with your nutritional doctor. I recommend one tablespoon of flaxseed oil two times a day or five to seven capsules two times a day.

Quercetin and other bioflavonoids like quercetin enhance the absorption of vitamin C and are found in foods such as citrus fruits, green tea and berries. Or one may take supplements of quercetin. Normally, for every 500 milligrams of vitamin C one should take at least 100 milligrams of quercetin or bioflavonoids.

As you have seen, certain vitamins and supplements can help your body win the battle against arthritis. Take hold of the things you can do in the natural, but don't forget the spiritual steps you can take as well.

Fighting Rheumatoid Arthritis

Nutritional supplements for rheumatoid arthritis

also include a multivitamin like Divine Health Multivitamins, which contain adequate amounts of B vitamins, minerals and antioxidants such as vitamins C and E.

Pantothenic acid is especially important, as well as B-complex vitamins. A dose of 2 grams a day may significantly reduce morning stiffness and pain.

Vitamin C and bioflavonoids also help reduce inflammation and histamine levels. I recommend 1000 milligrams of vitamin C three times a day. Many people are allergic to vitamin C since the majority of vitamin C comes from corn. Therefore, a patient with rheumatoid arthritis may need to be desensitized from corn in order to adequately absorb and utilize vitamin C. You can also find vitamin C buffered corn-free capsules in health food stores. Instead of deriving vitamin C from corn, these corn-free products derive vitamin C from such sources as the sago palm or beets.

Antioxidants are extremely important in overcoming rheumatoid arthritis. Take an antioxidant with a comprehensive antioxidant formula including vitamin C, beta carotene, vitamin E, selenium, n-acetyl-cysteine, lipoic acid, grape seed or pine bark extract and coenzyme Q_{10}. Grape seed extract and pine bark extract are particularly helpful with rheumatoid arthritis since they both help to relieve inflammation. You can find antioxidant capsules in health food stores.

I recommend 100 milligrams of grape seed or pine bark extract two times a day. The dose of vitamin C is 1,000 milligrams three times a day; vitamin E, 400 International Units one to two times a day; beta carotene, 25,000 units a day; selenium, 200 milligrams daily; n-acetyl-cysteine, 500 milligrams two times a day; lipoic acid, 100 milligrams daily and coenzyme Q_{10}, 50 milligrams two times a day.

MSM is high in sulfur. Taking at least 500 milligrams of MSM three times a day may help to alleviate the pain and swelling of rheumatoid arthritis.

Proteolytic enzymes may help to decrease inflammation. These enzymes usually have to be taken in a dose of four to five tablets, three times a day, between meals. However, you should be under the care of a nutritional doctor in order to manage this appropriately. If you have ulcer disease or inflammation of the stomach or duodenum, you should not take proteolytic enzymes.

Bromelain is an enzyme that comes from pineapple and is similar to proteolytic enzymes. It also has a potent anti-inflammatory effect. The normal dose is 500 milligrams, one to two tablets, three times a day between meals.

Curcumin comes from the yellow pigment of turmeric and has very strong anti-inflammatory properties. The normal dose of curcumin is 400 milligrams three times a day. Curcumin works especially well with bromelain when taken on an empty stomach.

Glucosamine sulfate is still the standard approach in nutritional therapy for rheumatoid arthritis, in a dose of 500–1000 milligrams three times a day. Glucosamine is a natural building block for the proteoglycans, one of the main components of cartilage.

> *My days are filled with grief . . . and my health is broken. I am exhausted and completely crushed. My groans come from an anguished heart. You know what I long for, Lord; you hear my every sigh.*
> —PSALM 38:6–9

Gamma oryzanol is a natural bran extract made from rice bran. You should take 100 milligrams three times a day. Often taken as a natural muscle builder, gamma oryzanol also helps to heal the intestinal lining.

L-glutamine helps to heal the intestinal lining. Take L-glutamine, 500 milligrams, ten to thirty minutes prior to meals. Also, taking the friendly bacteria, which is *lactobacillus acidophilus* and *bifidus,* helps to maintain a healthy intestinal environment in a dose of three billion colony-forming units per day.

Arthred, a low molecular-weight hydrolyzed collagen, is another very important nutrient for rebuilding cartilage. Collagen is the other main building block of cartilage, which is needed for the framework of the cartilage. I recommend 1 heaping tablespoon of arthred a day.

Chondroitin sulfate has been recommended in the past for treating both rheumatoid arthritis and osteoarthritis. However, chondroitin has very large molecules that are not well absorbed into the body when taken orally. Therefore, I have recommended that patients take glucosamine sulfate instead of chondroitin sulfate.

Ginger is an herb that has anti-inflammatory effects. A dose of approximately 4 grams of powdered ginger may be effective.

DHEA is a hormone that is usually low in people who suffer from rheumatoid arthritis. I obtain a DHEA level on all patients with rheumatoid arthritis, and then I supplement them with DHEA. A blood test by your nutritional doctor can help determine how much DHEA you may need.

Cetyl myristoleate is a fatty acid commonly found in beavers and sperm whales. It helps lubricate joints and reduce inflammation. A total dose of 1000 milligrams a day under the supervision of a nutritional doctor is recommended.

The typical treatments for rheumatoid arthritis are nonsteroidal, anti-inflammatory medications. These include naproxen and ibuprofen. However, this class of drugs can further damage your intestinal tract, leading to increased intestinal permeability or leaky gut (intestines). This leads to worsening of food allergies since our bodies absorbs whole food proteins.

In rheumatoid arthritis, the contrast to osteoarthritis is that you need to address the issues of poor digestion, increased intestinal permeability, food allergies and excessive inflammation. This needs to be done by a nutritional doctor. You may need an allergy desensitization diet, a comprehensive digestive stool analysis and supplementation in order to heal your intestinal tract.

In summary, the natural treatments of both rheumatoid arthritis and osteoarthritis are quite similar in that you should avoid the bad fat, such as animal fats and fried foods. You should eat the good fats, which are the fatty fish such as salmon and mackerel, and take flaxseed oil, as I mentioned earlier in this chapter.

Spiritual Exercise

Spiritually, reach out to your spiritual leaders and ask them to anoint you with oil and pray for you. Let the living water of Christ flow from your heart through your thoughts, feelings and emotions.

Because your body has been in pain, you may be tempted to make it the continual focus of your thoughts. Instead of thinking continually about your arthritic symptoms, decide to spend time thinking on this passage so that your body and mind will be renewed and refreshed daily:

> And so, dear Christian friends, I plead with you to give your bodies to God. Let them be a living and holy sacrifice—the kind he will accept. When you think of what he has done for you, is this too much to ask? Don't copy the behavior and customs of this world, but let God transform you into a new person by

changing the way you think. Then you will know what God wants you to do, and you will know how good and pleasing and perfect his will really is.

—ROMANS 12:1–2

Get Some Exercise

You should also *exercise* using both aerobic exercise and stretching exercises, which I will talk about in the next chapter.

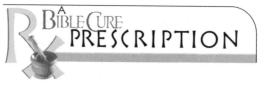

Overcoming Arthritis With
Vitamins and Supplements

List the first three steps you will take naturally to
overcome either your osteoarthritis or rheumatoid arthritis with vitamins and supplements:

1. _____

_____

_____

2. _____

_____

_____

3. _____

_____

_____

Ask the elders of your church to anoint you with
oil and pray for your healing.

Chapter 4

Overcoming Arthritis
With Exercise

While physical exercise may be painful at first, it is an essential ingredient in God's plan for you to overcome arthritis. Exercise not only decreases the risk of developing heart disease, cancer, hypertension, diabetes and osteoporosis, but it also decreases the risk of developing osteoarthritis. In other words, exercise helps prevent most degenerative diseases.

Do you already have osteoarthritis? Some exercises can actually worsen your condition, while others will greatly improve it. Do you have rheumatoid arthritis? Exercise can benefit you as well. Aquatic exercise can help both types of arthritis, because it is much easier on joints and muscles. Be sure to consult with your physician or physical therapist before starting any exercise program.

How does exercise help? Just as oil lubricates the moving parts of an engine, synovial fluid serves the function of lubricating cartilage. An adequate supply of synovial fluid will actually help prevent or slow down the development of osteoarthritis. Exercise helps to improve the flow of synovial fluid into and out of the cartilage. This in turn keeps the cartilage healthy and moist and prevents the drying and thinning of the cartilage that is so often seen in osteoarthritis. It is extremely important for the synovial fluid to keep the cartilage moist and wet in order to prevent frictional forces that dry out the cartilage and cause wear and tear and thinning.

Exercising also helps you lose weight. One of the best preventive measures for osteoarthritis is reaching your ideal or normal body weight. As I said earlier, obesity and excess body weight are associated with increased stress on the weight-bearing joints, which will eventually trigger osteoarthritis. I'll give you some practical advice on how to lose weight through exercise later in this Bible Cure booklet.

I know that losing weight is more than just a physical issue. It's so important that you seek God's help to overcome any desire to overeat. Remember the promise of Scripture: "For I can do everything with the help of Christ who gives me the strength I need" (Phil. 4:13).

A BIBLE CURE HEALTH TIP

Take these spiritual steps right now:

- Ask God to break any food addiction or eating disorder that afflicts you.
- Seek the Spirit's guidance for selecting someone to help hold you accountable for your eating habits.
- Accept God's desire and provision to supply all your needs, including your physical needs for food.

While there are variables that may affect your ideal weight, the guidelines found in these height and weight tables are helpful for knowing if you may be overweight.[1]

Height and Weight Table for Women

Height	Small Frame	Medium Frame	Large Frame
4'10"	102–111 lbs.	109–121 lbs.	118–131 lbs.
4'11"	103–113 lbs.	111–123 lbs.	120–134 lbs.
5'0"	104–115 lbs.	113–126 lbs.	122–137 lbs.
5'1"	106–118 lbs.	115–129 lbs.	125–140 lbs.
5'2"	108–121 lbs.	118–132 lbs.	128–143 lbs.
5'3"	111–124 lbs.	121–135 lbs.	131–147 lbs.
5'4"	114–127 lbs.	124–138 lbs.	134–151 lbs.
5'5"	117–130 lbs.	127–141 lbs.	137–155 lbs.
5'6"	120–133 lbs.	130–144 lbs.	140–159 lbs.
5'7"	123–136 lbs.	133–147 lbs.	143–163 lbs.
5'8"	126–139 lbs.	136–150 lbs.	146–167 lbs.
5'9"	129–142 lbs.	139–153 lbs.	149–170 lbs.
5'10"	132–145 lbs.	142–156 lbs.	152–173 lbs.
5'11"	135–148 lbs.	145–159 lbs.	155–176 lbs.
6'0"	138–151 lbs.	148–162 lbs.	158–179 lbs.

Height and Weight Table for Men

Height	Small Frame	Medium Frame	Large Frame
5'2"	128–134 lbs.	131–141 lbs.	138–150 lbs.
5'3"	130–136 lbs.	133–143 lbs.	140–153 lbs.
5'4"	132–138 lbs.	135–145 lbs.	142–156 lbs.
5'5"	134–140 lbs.	137–148 lbs.	144–160 lbs.
5'6"	136–142 lbs.	139–151 lbs.	146–164 lbs.
5'7"	138–145 lbs.	142–154 lbs.	149–168 lbs.
5'8"	140–148 lbs.	145–157 lbs.	152–172 lbs.
5'9"	142–151 lbs.	148–160 lbs.	155–176 lbs.
5'10"	144–154 lbs.	151–163 lbs.	158–180 lbs.
5'11"	146–157 lbs.	154–166 lbs.	161–184 lbs.
6'0"	149–160 lbs.	157–170 lbs.	164–188 lbs.
6'1"	152–164 lbs.	160–174 lbs.	168–192 lbs.
6'2"	155–168 lbs.	164–178 lbs.	172–197 lbs.
6'3"	158–172 lbs.	167–182 lbs.	176–202 lbs.
6'4"	162–176 lbs.	171–187 lbs.	181–207 lbs.

When you exercise, use a heart rate monitor. Prior to beginning an aerobic exercise program you will want to purchase a heart rate monitor and should calculate your training heart rate.

Train within your heart rate zone. To compute this, subtract your age from 220, and then multiply this number times .65. Repeat the process, but multiply that number times .80.

> *Oh, the joys of those who are kind to the poor. The LORD rescues them in times of trouble . . . The LORD nurses them when they are sick and eases their pain and discomfort. "O LORD," I prayed, "have mercy on me. Heal me, for I have sinned against you."*
> —PSALM 41:1–4

220 minus [your age] = _____
times 0.65 = _____

220 minus [your age] = _____
times 0.80 = _____

The range between the two numbers is the range for which you should be aiming.

Drink adequate water. Adequate hydration and exercise are probably the two most important components in assuring adequate flow of the synovial fluid into and out of the cartilage.

Maintain the range of motion of joints. Exercise also helps maintain the range of motion of a joint. The less a joint is used, the less range of motion you will maintain. An example of this is when a patient develops a painful shoulder and will not use the shoulder. He will not reach overhead or exercise the shoulder through a full range of motion. Within one to three weeks, he may develop a frozen shoulder and be unable to extend his arm overhead or adequately rotate his shoulder. By not using the shoulder on a daily basis, he will actually lose the function of the shoulder. In other words, exercise maintains the flexibility of the joint. Avoidance of exercise can severely limit the normal range of motion of a joint.

Strengthen your tendons, ligaments and muscles. Exercise also strengthens the tendons, ligaments and muscles that support the joint. This in turn adds more protection for the joint. Well-developed and well-toned muscles, tendons and ligaments help to protect the joints by absorbing the majority of the force placed on the joints.

Each time you exercise, you put pressure on the joints. The majority of the pressure is absorbed by the supporting structures, including the muscles, ligaments and tendons.

Since cartilage has no blood vessels, the cartilage relies on an exchange of fluid through the synovial fluid in order to take in nutrients and eliminate waste products. Exercise encourages this process of taking in nutrients into the cartilage through the synovial fluid and expelling waste products or toxic material out of the cartilage.

> *I am suffering and in pain. Rescue me, O God, by your saving power. Then I will praise God's name with singing, and I will honor him with thanksgiving.*
> —PSALM 69:29–30

Weight-bearing exercises are some of the best forms of exercise for arthritis sufferers. However, if arthritis is severe, you should start with nonweight-bearing exercises and gradually work into weight-bearing exercises. Weight-bearing exercises are simply exercises, such as walking, low-impact aerobics and stair-stepper, where you are actually working against the force of gravity. Weight-bearing exercises help the bones grow stronger and thicker. However, this form of exercise is most effective for the lower part of the body, especially the ankles, knees, hips and lower back, more so than the upper body.

Weightlifting and other isotonic types of exercises are also important in helping to build strong bones and muscles. You should lift light weights at very slow speeds and perform at least eight to twelve repetitions a set. To avoid injury, seek a certified personal trainer to instruct you on the proper techniques in lifting weights.

Walking. Patients who have moderate to severe arthritis are often unable to walk sufficient distances to adequately work the muscles. Therefore, for these patients I recommend alternative aerobic-type exercises. These include cycling, gliding machines such as the Precor machine and water aerobics. These exercises take most of the strain off the joints while at the same time strengthening the supporting structures, tendons and ligaments and stimulating the flow of the synovial fluid in the joints.

Prior to beginning an aerobic exercise program, you should be screened by your medical doctor in order to rule out significant cardiovascular disease. I recommend that my arthritis patients perform aerobic exercise three to four times a week for at least twenty minutes.

Often arthritis patients are only able to start out at five minutes each time; gradually they can work up to twenty minutes by increasing the amount of exercise every week or two. I have seen so many of my patients who have begun to exercise on a regular basis improve to such an extent that I am able to decrease or eliminate their medications entirely.

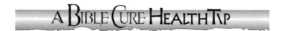

A BIBLE CURE HEALTH TIP

Four Important Steps
for Overcoming Osteoarthritis

- Drink two to three quarts of purified water daily for adequate hydration.
- Do regular aerobic exercise.
- Take glucosamine sulfate with adequate water consumption.
- Achieve ideal body weight.

The importance of stretching. Stretching exercises are also very important for both preventing arthritis and improving flexibility in arthritic joints. In starting an exercise program, it is best to warm up for five to ten minutes on a stationary bike, gliding machine or treadmill. After you have adequately warmed your muscles up, then stretch anywhere from ten to twenty minutes. Stretching increases your flexibility, improves the range of motion of a joint and makes you less prone to injury during weight-lifting exercises.

After stretching, lift weights for approximately twenty to thirty minutes. I recommend weight machines rather free weights since you would be less prone to injure yourself with the machines. After working out with weights, then perform aerobic exercise such as cycling, gliding, stair-stepper or walking on the treadmill for twenty minutes at your training heart rate.

After completing this, have a five-minute cooldown in which you walk at a slower speed. Then stretch slowly and hold the movement at the end of the stretch for approximately one to two seconds. If you develop pain in the joint, stop stretching in this manner. Count one, one thousand, two, one thousand, and then release the stretch. Perform anywhere from ten to twenty repetitions per movement. Some basic stretches include neck, back, knee, hip and leg stretches.

Your Bible Cure prescription for overcoming arthritis includes regular exercise of your faith and your body. Don't give up and sit around nursing your pain. Take positive actions and think positive, faith-filled thoughts today. You can overcome arthritis when you take care of your body and exercise your faith boldly through prayer.

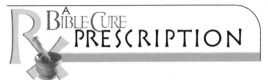

BIBLE CURE PRESCRIPTION

Overcoming Arthritis
With Exercise

Check the steps you will take daily:

❏ Maintain an ideal body weight.

❏ Drink enough water—two to three quarts
of water a day.

❏ Do aerobic exercise and stretching—at
least four times a week.

❏ Exercise your faith by boldly approaching
God's throne in prayer, seeking His healing for your arthritis.

Chapter 5

Overcoming Negative Thoughts and Emotions

T he Bible cure affirms the benefits of both physical and spiritual exercise for our continuing health. "Physical exercise has some value, but spiritual exercise is much more important, for it promises a reward in both this life and the next. This is true, and everyone should accept it" (1 Tim. 4:8–9). As you exercise your faith, trusting God to remove pain, strengthen and heal your body, you will boldly pray for your healing.

I have explained to you the physical benefits of exercise in overcoming arthritis; now let me share with you the spiritual benefits of exercising your faith and boldly praying for your healing. God's Word encourages us:

So let us come boldly to the throne of

our gracious God. There we will receive
his mercy, and we will find grace to help
us when we need it.

—Hebrews 4:16

You can boldly approach God's throne in
prayer. How?

- Believe in faith, trusting God the Healer for
  your healing.
- Trust His promises to heal you; for example, "He [God] sent his word, and healed
  them, and delivered them from their de-
  structions" (Ps. 107:20, kjv).
- Pray boldly for your healing, knowing that
  in His mercy and grace, God's will for you
  is to walk in divine health.

A Bible Cure Prayer
FOR YOU

*Almighty God, in the name of Jesus and
through His shed blood, I boldly approach
Your throne of grace and seek Your heal-
ing power and touch. I know that by
Jesus' stripes I have been healed. I claim
Your promise that You have forgiven all*

*my sins and healed all my diseases. So I
boldly stand on Your promises of healing,
and I praise You for helping me to overcome arthritis in my body. In the name of
Jesus, amen.*

Extinguish Negative Thoughts and Emotions

Negative emotions stifle faith and inhibit the
body's ability to receive healing. In 1993, the
National Institute for Healthcare Research in
Rockville, Maryland, compiled hundreds of studies on the health benefits of faith. Their report was
called "The Faith Factor." The NIHR discovered
that 77 percent of the studies on the relationship
between faith and illness demonstrated that faith
had a positive effect, increasing people's general
health and their survival rates.[1]

In this Bible cure for arthritis, I believe that we
must also address the emotional issues in our
lives that may inhibit both faith and healing. I have
observed that many patients with rheumatoid
arthritis have negative emotions. These harmful
negative emotions can intensify and aggravate the

symptoms of arthritis. Circle any of these emotions that you may have:

Anger	Bitterness	Guilt
Resentment	Shame	Hatred
Fear	Anxiety	Depression

I will never forget one patient that I had about ten years ago. When I initially saw her, she was approximately forty-five years old. At that time she appeared to be the picture of health with no joint pains or any other illnesses.

However, she had just gone through a divorce. She began to hold so much bitterness and resentment toward her husband that I watched her over the following ten years become crippled with arthritis. She began having deformities of her hands, fingers, knees and toes.

> *Jesus . . . healed people who had every kind of sickness and disease . . . whatever their illness and pain, or if they were possessed by demons, or were epileptics, or were paralyzed he healed them all.*
> —MATTHEW 4:23–24

Despite all my efforts, and the efforts of one of the top rheumatologists in town, this woman's arthritis continued to worsen. I believe it was due to the harmful emotions of bitterness, resentment and hatred that she had for her ex-husband. It is, therefore, critically important for all sufferers of rheumatoid arthritis to forgive whoever has wronged them.

You cannot simply do a mental forgiveness. This will not stop the process. You need a Holy Spirit-led, deep forgiveness in order to break these deadly emotions of anger, resentment and hatred that can cripple your body. I believe that "a merry heart doeth good like a medicine: but a broken spirit drieth the bones" (Prov. 17:22, KJV). I believe that "a broken spirit drieth the bones" actually means that one can develop arthritis.

> *And even we Christians, although we have the Holy Spirit within us as a foretaste of future glory, also groan to be released from pain and suffering. We, too, wait anxiously for that day when God will give us our full rights as his children, including the new bodies he has promised us.*
> —ROMANS 8:23

Your mental attitudes and emotions must be controlled by your faith in Christ. You cannot succumb to your negative attitudes or bad feelings. If you do, arthritis will begin to overcome you. Instead, be an overcomer. Overcome the painful disease of arthritis by choosing faith over doubt, hope over discouragement and, most of all, God's healing promises over the debilitating effects of arthritis. You are an overcomer, and your disease has already been defeated at the cross of Christ!

Overcoming Negative Emotions

Take these steps toward eliminating negative thoughts and emotions, strengthening your faith, building hope and opening your life up to the healing power of God.

Step 1—Take daily doses of God's Word.
Read these scriptures aloud three times a day, especially before meals and at bedtime to break any strongholds over your body and mind.

Overcoming anger—Ephesians 4:26–27
Overcoming bitterness—Ephesians 4:31–32
Overcoming guilt—Psalm 103:11–13
Overcoming resentment—Romans 12:19–21
Overcoming shame—Isaiah 49:23
Overcoming hatred—Matthew 5:43–44
Overcoming fear—2 Timothy 1:7
Overcoming anxiety—Philippians 4:6–7

Step 2—Pray boldly in faith.

Don't be timid about claiming God's promises for your healing and health. Trust His Word.

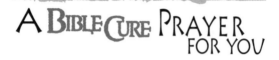

A BIBLE CURE PRAYER
FOR YOU

Almighty God, You are the God who heals. I ask for Your healing power to restore health to my joints and aching bones. I seek Your healing balm for my arthritis, and I ask that You send forth Your Word and heal my body. Take away all stiffness, soreness, swelling, pain and aching through the precious blood of Jesus. You are Jehovah Rapha, the God who Heals. I claim Your healing power in my life. In Jesus' name and for His glory, I am healed. Amen.

Step 3—Begin praising God for His healing power at work in you.

What does the Bible say about praising God? Do as the psalmist declares:

I will praise the LORD at all times. I will constantly speak his praises. I will boast only in the LORD; let all who are discouraged take heart. Come, let us tell of the LORD'S greatness; let us exalt his name together. I prayed to the LORD, and he answered me, freeing me from all my fears. Those who look to him for help will be radiant with joy; no shadow of shame will darken their faces. I cried out to the LORD in my suffering, and he heard me. He set me free from all my fears.

—PSALMS 34:1–6

How do you praise God continually? Remember to praise Him based on His promises not your circumstances. Praise Him for your healing already purchased at the cross through His shed blood:

He personally carried away our sins in his own body on the cross so we can be dead to sin and live for what is right. You have been healed by his wounds!

—1 PETER 2:24

It's now time to trust His Word, receive His healing, cast out negative thoughts and emotions and praise God for His healing power at work in your life. Begin praising Him today—and don't stop!

R℞ BIBLE CURE PRESCRIPTION

1. Take daily doses of God's Word.

Check each of the following boxes to indicate your commitment to overcome that emotion:

❑ Anger—Ephesians 4:26–27
❑ Bitterness—Ephesians 4:31–32
❑ Guilt—Psalm 103:11–13
❑ Resentment—Romans 12:19–21
❑ Shame—Isaiah 49:23
❑ Hatred—Matthew 5:43–44
❑ Fear—2 Timothy 1:7
❑ Anxiety—Philippians 4:6–7

2. Pray boldly in faith.

Write a prayer, boldly claiming God's promises to you that will lead to healing and health in these areas:

_____

_____

3. Now praise God for His healing power in you.

Notes

PREFACE
YOU CAN OVERCOME ARTHRITIS

1. Burton Goldberg Group, *Alternative Medicine, The Definitive Guide* (Puyallup, WA: Fullness Medicine Publishing, Inc., 1993), 532.

CHAPTER 2
OVERCOMING ARTHRITIS WITH
PROPER NUTRITION

1. Ariza-Ariza, R, et al. Ref: Seminars in Arthritis and Rheumatism. 1998; 27:366–370.
2. Ibid.
3. You can read more about this therapy in Dr. Nambudripad's book, *Say Goodbye to Illness.* One may find this resource by looking under N.A.E.T. on the Internet at www.naet.com.
4. Selene Yeager, et al, *New Foods for Healing (*Emmaus, PA: Rodale Press, 1998), 171.

CHAPTER 3
OVERCOMING ARTHRITIS WITH
VITAMINS AND SUPPLEMENTS

1. Internet source from www.drmorrow.com.
2. A. L Vaz, "Double-blind clinical evaluation of the relative efficacy of ibuprofen and glucosamine sulfate in the management of osteoarthritis of the knee in outpatients." *Curr. Med. Res. Opin.,* 8:145–9, 1982.

3. Adapted from E. D'Ambrosio, et al., "Glucosamine Sulfate: A Controlled Clinical Investigation in Arthrosis," *Pharmatherapeutica*, v. 2, p. 504, 1981.

CHAPTER 4
OVERCOMING ARTHRITIS WITH EXERCISE

1. Obtained from Internet source, www.heartscreen.com.

CHAPTER 5
OVERCOMING NEGATIVE THOUGHTS AND EMOTIONS

1. Koenig, Harold G. *The Healing Power of Faith: Science Explores Medicine's Last Great Frontier* (New York: Simon & Schuster, 1999), 258.

Don Colbert, M.D., was born in Tupelo, Mississippi. He attended Oral Roberts School of Medicine in Tulsa, Oklahoma, where he received a bachelor of science degree in biology in addition to his degree in medicine. Dr. Colbert completed his internship and residency with Florida Hospital in Orlando, Florida. He is board certified in family practice and has received extensive training in nutritional medicine.

If you would like more
information about natural and
divine healing, or information about
Divine Health Nutritional Products®,
you may contact
Dr. Colbert at:

DR. DON COLBERT

1908 Boothe Circle
Longwood, FL 32750
Telephone: 407-331-7007

Dr. Colbert's website is
www.drcolbert.com.

BIBLE CURE

NOTES

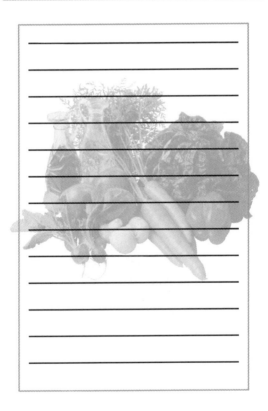

_____
_____
_____
_____
_____
_____
_____
_____
_____
_____
_____
_____

BIBLE CURE

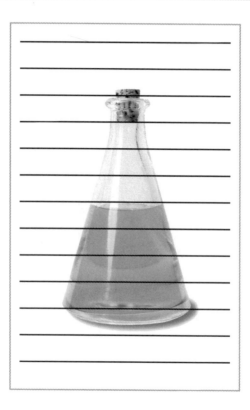

BIBLE CURE

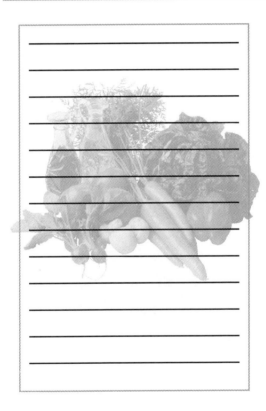

BIBLE CURE

NOTES

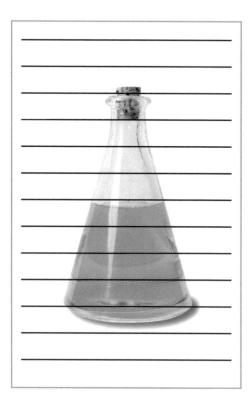

BIBLE CURE

NOTES

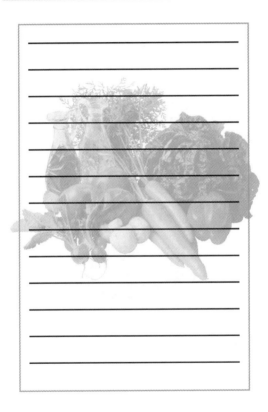

_____
_____
_____
_____
_____
_____
_____
_____
_____
_____
_____
_____
_____

BIBLE CURE

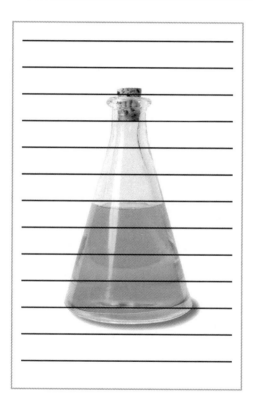

BIBLE CURE

NOTES

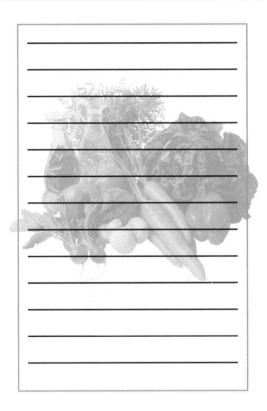

_____
_____
_____
_____
_____
_____
_____
_____
_____
_____
_____
_____
_____

BIBLE CURE

NOTES

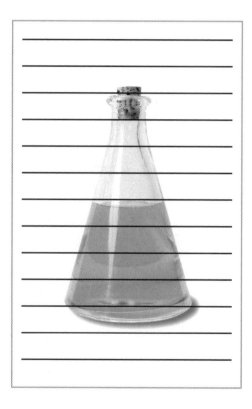

_____
_____
_____
_____
_____
_____
_____
_____
_____
_____
_____
_____
_____

BIBLE CURE

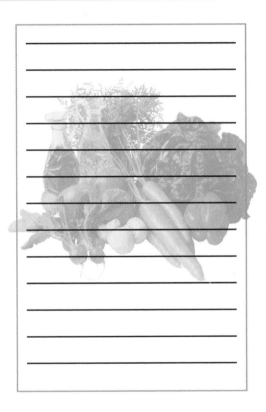

_____
_____
_____
_____
_____
_____
_____
_____
_____
_____
_____
_____
_____

Pick up these other Siloam Press
books by Dr. Colbert:

Toxic Relief
Walking in Divine Health
What You Don't Know May Be Killing You

The Bible Cure® Booklet Series

The Bible Cure for ADD and Hyperactivity
The Bible Cure for Allergies
The Bible Cure for Arthritis
The Bible Cure for Cancer
The Bible Cure for Candida and Yeast Infection
The Bible Cure for Chronic Fatigue and Fibromyalgia
The Bible Cure for Depression and Anxiety
The Bible Cure for Diabetes
The Bible Cure for Headaches
The Bible Cure for Heart Disease
The Bible Cure for Heartburn and Indigestion
The Bible Cure for High Blood Pressure
The Bible Cure for Memory Loss
The Bible Cure for Menopause
The Bible Cure for Osteoporosis
The Bible Cure for PMS and Mood Swings
The Bible Cure for Sleep Disorders
The Bible Cure for Weight Loss and Muscle Gain

SILOAM PRESS

A part of Strang Communications Company
600 Rinehart Road
Lake Mary, FL 34726
(800) 599-5750